DRUGS AND MENTAL ILLNESS

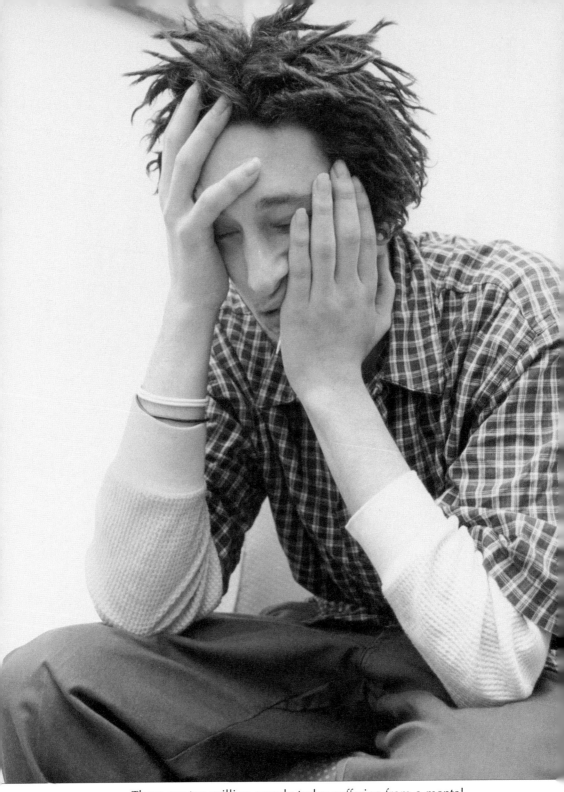

There are ten million people today suffering from a mental health disorder who also abuse or are addicted to drugs.

THE DRUG ABUSE PREVENTION LIBRARY

DRUGS AND MENTAL ILLNESS

Maia Miller

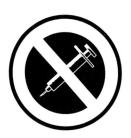

THE ROSEN PUBLISHING GROUP, INC.
NEW YORK

Published in 2000 by The Rosen Publishing Group, Inc.
29 East 21st Street, New York, NY 10010

Library of Congress Cataloging-in-Publication Data

Miller, Maia
    Drugs and mental illness / Maia Miller
        p. cm. — (The drug abuse prevention library)
    Includes bibliographical references and index.
    Summary: Discusses the relationship between drugs and mental illness and shows how drugs and addiction cause irrational behavior and promote personality disorders.
    ISBN 0-8239-3155-2 (lib. bdg.)
        1. Narcotics addicts—Mental health—Juvenile literature. 2. Mentally ill—Substance abuse—Juvenile literature. [1. Drug abuse. 2. Mentally ill.] I. Title. II. Series.
RC564.3 .M55 2000
616.86—dc21   99-046390

Manufactured in the United States of America

Contents

	Introduction	7
Chapter 1	The Dangers of Drugs	13
Chapter 2	What Drugs Are Out There?	20
Chapter 3	Drug-Induced Mental Illness	30
Chapter 4	Teens, Drugs, and the Mind	41
Chapter 5	Drugs That Help	48
	Glossary	57
	Where to Go for Help	59
	For Further Reading	61
	Index	62

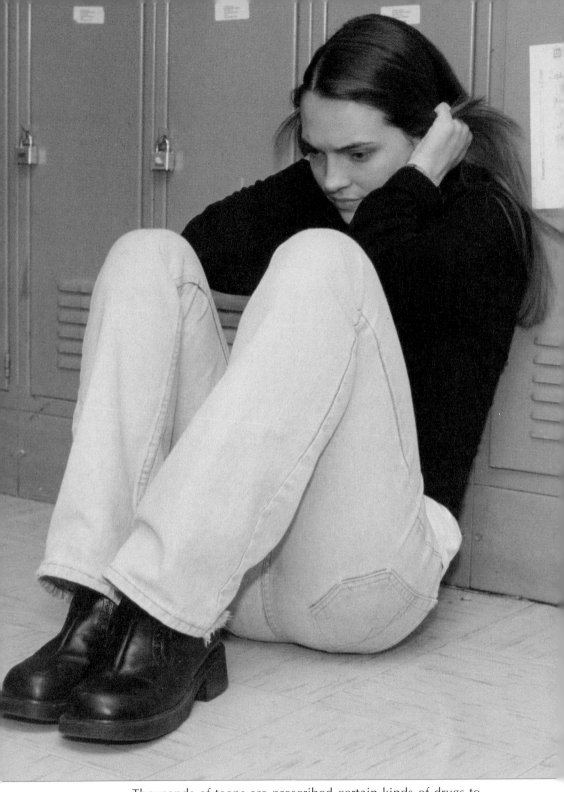
Thousands of teens are prescribed certain kinds of drugs to deal with mental illnesses such as depression.

Introduction

Marnie giggled, then took another long drag of the joint that was being passed around. She closed her eyes, feeling the drug take effect. Everything was slow and relaxed. Her parents' divorce, her breakup with Max, the fight with her mother that morning—like the one they had every morning—all of that seemed miles away.

Marnie's friend Jade had introduced her to pot a few months ago, over winter break. Marnie had been really nervous at first, but after smoking a few times, she had begun to look forward to using it. Now she was getting stoned almost every day. She was falling behind in her classes, and sometimes she had to steal from her mother's wallet to pay for the drugs, but Marnie didn't care.

8

When Darnell joined the track team in ninth grade, he had high hopes of following in his brother Jared's footsteps. Jared had been the top athlete on the team and last year had won a track scholarship to go to a local college.

At the end of his first season, however, Darnell's times were still just average—and way below Jared's. Darnell decided to go on a rigorous diet and training schedule, eating only raw vegetables and plain rice and running five to six miles a day. When his mother finally brought him to a doctor several months later, Darnell had lost almost forty pounds.

The doctor sent him to a psychiatrist, who diagnosed Darnell with anorexia. She prescribed Prozac, an antidepressant medication that would help Darnell both with his eating disorder and with some of the other problems he was having. After six months of medication and therapy, Darnell was eating regularly and was able to express some of his frustrations through words instead of self-destructive behavior.

Noriko is sixteen. She has been addicted to heroin for over two years—almost as long as she has been a prostitute. Noriko ran away from home two years ago because her stepfather was sexually abusing her. The man who found her sleeping in the park offered her food, shelter, and kindness at first, but then demanded that Noriko sell her body to pay him back. He also got her addicted to heroin.

Now Noriko spends most of her time shooting heroin or selling her body to earn enough money to buy more drugs. If she goes for more than two days without heroin, Noriko suffers severe nausea, chills, sweating, and stomach cramps.

These three teens' stories reflect the wide variety of ways that drugs and mental illness can be interconnected. As you can see, the relationship between mental problems and drugs—illegal street drugs and prescription medicines—is very complicated.

You might be expecting this book to tell you that drugs are always bad for your body and brain. However, the truth is that millions of people around the world use certain kinds of drugs to improve both their physical and mental health. Think about Darnell's case for a moment. With the help of an anti-depressant drug, Darnell was able to overcome some of the negative feelings he had about himself and was able to change his self-destructive eating habits.

Unfortunately, more often the connection between drugs and mental illness in teenagers

10 is not a healthy one. Like many teens, Marnie uses drugs as an attempt to escape her unhappy feelings. In reality, however, she is only making the situation worse.

Noriko is beyond the experimentation stage of drug use; she is addicted. That means that along with any emotional problems that her stepfather's abuse may have caused, Noriko has two additional mental disorders: drug abuse and drug addiction.

There are ten million people today suffering from a mental health disorder who also abuse or are addicted to drugs. Add in the parents, siblings, and close friends of these individuals and you have got an estimated forty million people whose lives are affected by mental illness and drug problems.

This large number makes it especially important to understand drug abuse and mental health and to find out more about how they interact. Doctors who treat patients with both drug-related problems and mental illness frequently correctly diagnose one condition but not the other. This often makes effective treatment very difficult.

This book provides an introduction to drugs—how they are used, who uses them, and what effects they have—as well as a discussion of some of the mental illnesses that

are most commonly associated with drug | *11*
use. If you think that you or someone you
know may be suffering from drug problems,
mental illness, or both, read on to gain a
better understanding of these complex conditions. You could be saving a life.

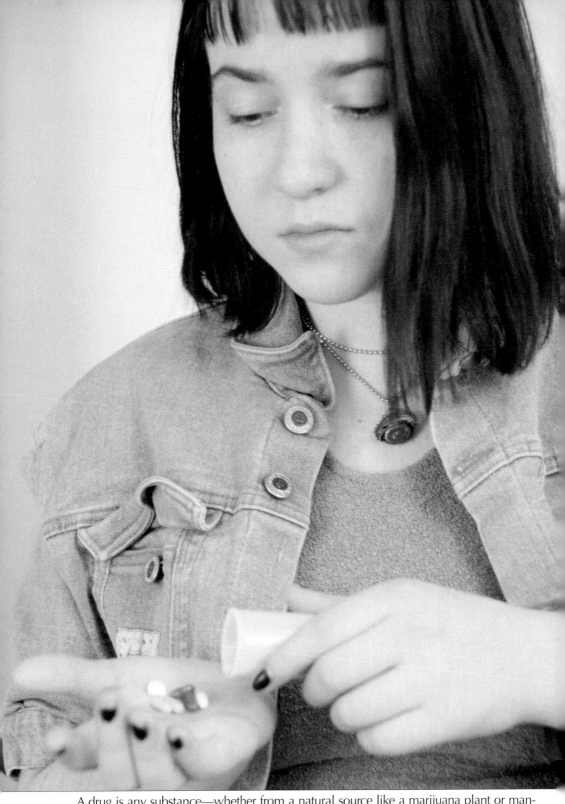

A drug is any substance—whether from a natural source like a marijuana plant or man-made such as a prescription medication—that changes how you think, feel, or act.

CHAPTER 1

The Dangers of Drugs

To get a better picture of how drugs and mental illness go hand in hand, a good working knowledge of what drugs are and how they work is vital.

Defining Drugs

A drug is any substance—whether from a natural source or man-made—that changes how you think, feel, or act. The two drugs that cause the most suffering in the United States, alcohol and nicotine (found in cigarettes and chewing tobacco), are legal. Drugs that require a prescription, such as allergy medications, penicillin, and antidepressants, are also legal, although some of these substances are used illegally. Over-the-counter (OTC) medications, like aspirin, cough syrup, and stay-awake

13

14 drugs, are available in supermarkets and pharmacies and can be purchased without a prescription.

Some potentially dangerous drugs can be found in common foods and drinks. Coffee, tea, soda, and chocolate, for instance, contain caffeine. In addition, certain household products, such as glue and cleaning supplies, can be used incorrectly to produce druglike effects on the body.

You might think that if a drug is available in a supermarket and can be bought by anyone, it must be safe. That is simply not true. Any drug can be harmful—legal drugs that are taken in too large dosages or for too long a time, medications used without a prescription, and illegal drugs used to get high.

Abuse and Addiction

Before looking at specific types of drugs, let's define a few key ideas. You have probably heard the terms "drug abuse" and "drug addiction" before. But do you know the difference between them?

Drug Abuse

Most professionals in the mental health field—including psychologists, psychiatrists, social workers, and researchers—use a book called the *Diagnostic and Statistical Manual of Mental Disorders,*

Fourth Edition (DSM-IV) to define and diagnose a wide variety of mental illnesses. The *DSM-IV* defines drug abuse as using a drug so much that its effects seriously damage the person's health and his or her performance at school or on the job.

Drug Addiction

Like drug abuse, drug addiction involves the continued use of drugs despite significant substance-related problems. Unlike drug abuse, however, addiction means that the user is physically or psychologically dependent on the drug in order to feel and act normal. Cocaine addicts cannot use cocaine only once a month at parties and feel normal on other days. They have a craving for the drug almost all the time and feel both mentally and physically sick when none is available.

The main characteristics of drug addiction that make it different from drug abuse are tolerance, withdrawal, and a pattern of compulsive use. Let's examine what these terms mean.

- *Tolerance:* If you continue to take drugs, your body soon develops a tolerance to them. This means that you

16

need to use more and more of the drug to get the desired effect. The longer a person takes drugs and the more he or she uses them, the higher his or her tolerance will be.

• *Withdrawal:* When someone uses drugs frequently, his or her body becomes accustomed to the substance. When drug use is suddenly stopped, the body goes into withdrawal. Noriko's story in the introduction to this book describes some typical withdrawal symptoms: nausea, sweating, cramps, and chills. Other common signs are depression, insomnia (the inability to sleep), and confusion.

• *Compulsive use:* Someone who is addicted to drugs feels a compulsion, or an extremely strong need, to use them, even though he or she knows that the drug use is causing significant physical or psychological problems.

Two Kinds of Addiction

There are two aspects to drug addiction: physical addiction and psychological addiction. Both of these elements make it very difficult for addicts to stop using drugs.

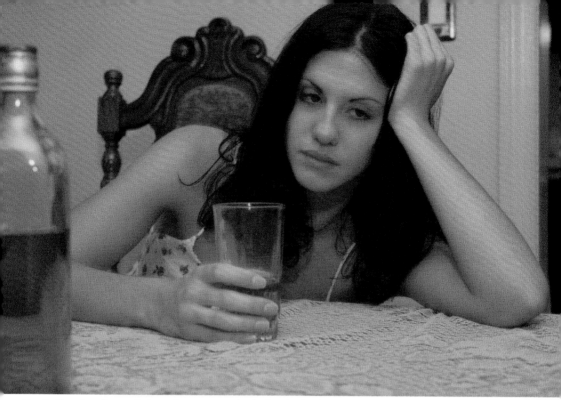

Alcoholics develop cellular tolerance to alcohol, which changes the way the brain works, and when they stop drinking, they cannot immediately return to their normal balanced state.

Physical Addiction

When someone uses a drug very frequently, actual physical and chemical changes occur in his or her body and brain in reaction to the presence of the drug. This means that the user craves the drug not just out of habit, but also because his or her body now needs the drug to function normally.

A physical change that occurs in the body of alcoholics is called cellular tolerance. This involves a change in the way the brain works. In general, messages are sent from the body to the brain and vice versa by way of cells in the brain called neurons. In the brain of a heavy alcohol drinker,

17

18 | certain neurons send messages much faster than the same neurons in a nonaddict. When someone addicted to alcohol suddenly stops drinking, his or her brain cannot immediately return to its normal balanced state.

Psychological Addiction

Psychological addiction happens when a drug user becomes addicted to the way that he or she feels when high on the drug. For instance, an amphetamine addict might crave the huge burst of energy that he or she feels from using speed.

When someone is psychologically addicted to drugs, the thought of drugs is always on his or her mind. The person's life revolves largely around using the drug or finding ways to get it. Usually this stems from the person's false belief that drugs can help that person cope with stress, sadness, or fear.

Is There a Problem?

Do you think that you or someone you know may have a problem with drugs? Here are some common warning signs:

- Mood swings
- Loss of interest in activities, such as sports, clubs, or hobbies

- Feelings of worthlessness and hopelessness
- Poor grades or skipping school
- Hanging out with a new group of friends known for risky behavior
- Parents who use drugs or who are easygoing about their children experimenting with drugs
- Family history of abuse or addiction to drugs
- History of physical, emotional, or sexual abuse

If three or more of these sound familiar, you could have a serious problem. The sooner the problem is identified and treated, the better the chance of recovery.

If you think you might have a drug problem, have hope. The truth is that there is help out there, and it can make you feel good about yourself. You can live your life without drugs. There are organizations listed in the back of this book that can help get you on the path to recovery. Once you start living a drug-free life, you will see that the best highs come from finding an activity that is challenging and rewarding. Drugs offer nothing more than empty promises.

CHAPTER 2

What Drugs Are Out There?

Medications

When used properly, medications, which are available both over-the-counter and by prescription, safely help millions of people every day to feel better. Widely used medications include aspirin, cold medicines, nasal sprays, and antacids.

Some medications are used illegally, without a prescription, to get high. Common examples are Xanax and Valium, which in low doses reduce anxiety and make people feel extremely relaxed but in larger doses can cause mild euphoria (extreme happiness).

When used in the wrong dosage, by the wrong person, or in combination with certain other substances, however, legal medications can be just as dangerous as street drugs.

Alcohol

Excluding cigarette smoking, alcoholism (the abusive use of alcohol) is by far the most serious drug problem in the United States, affecting millions of Americans. Although selling alcohol to anyone under twenty-one is illegal, many teens have access to it.

Alcohol is usually the first drug that teens try, and many are unaware of its harmful effects. One particularly dangerous trend among teens and college students is binge drinking, which involves consuming huge amounts of alcohol in a short period of time and can result in coma and death.

In small to medium doses, alcohol makes most people more talkative, more outgoing, and less inhibited (shy or awkward) around other people. Because of these effects, many people think of alcohol as a stimulant. However, alcohol is actually a depressant, also known as a downer. Higher doses of alcohol can cause slowed and impaired speech and movement; problems with vision, taste, and smell; and decreased reflex responses. Memory problems are also a common effect; short-term memory is

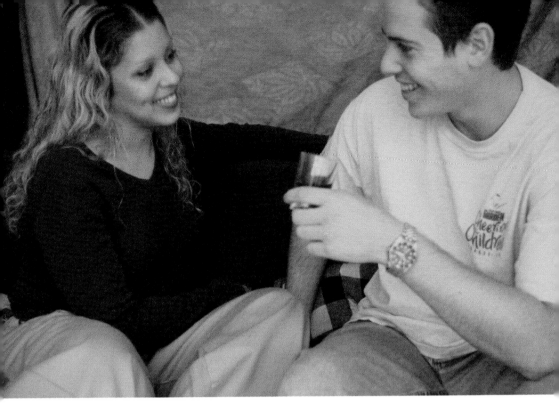

Alcohol is usually the first drug that teens try, and many are unaware of its harmful effects.

reduced, and heavy drinkers may experience blackouts, or periods of time when they have no memory of the events surrounding the drinking episode.

Cocaine, Amphetamines, and Other Stimulants

Stimulants include street drugs such as cocaine, crack, and amphetamines, as well as prescription drugs such as Benzedrine and Dexedrine. In general, stimulants heighten alertness, decrease appetite and the need for sleep, and create extremely pleasurable feelings. Among twelfth-graders interviewed for a 1998 study,

cocaine was the most commonly used stim- | *23*
ulant (9.3 percent), followed by amphetamines (7.1 percent).

One of the most addictive drugs known today, cocaine is generally sold on the street as a white crystalline powder that is snorted, swallowed, or sometimes made into a liquid to be injected. Common street names for cocaine include coke, C, snow, sugar, flake, and blow. Within minutes of taking the drug, most users feel euphoric, talkative, energetic, and mentally alert. Physical symptoms include rapid heartbeat and breathing and raised blood pressure and body temperature.

In large doses and over long periods of time, the effects of cocaine can be extremely dangerous: chest pain, nausea, blurred vision, fever, convulsions, coma, and death. Users who have taken cocaine for a long time lose the euphoric feeling and instead experience the drug's far less pleasant long-term effects: restlessness, mood swings, loss of interest in sex, insomnia, paranoia, hallucinations, and delusions (see chapter 3).

Street amphetamines, often called speed, crank, and uppers, can be sniffed, smoked, injected, or eaten. Their effects on users are similar to those of cocaine: euphoria and alertness, lack of appetite, rapid breathing

24 | and heart rate, blurred vision, and fever. At high doses, amphetamines can lead to tremors (severe shaking), loss of coordination, collapse, and death due to heart failure or extremely high fever. Long-term amphetamine use can cause violent and irrational behavior and even psychosis (severe hallucinations and an inability to tell what is real and what is imaginary).

Depressants (Sedative-Hypnotics)

Depressants, also known as sedative-hypnotics, are among the most popular drugs in the United States and are very addictive. The two main classes of depressants are barbiturates and benzodiazepines. In general, depressants slow down the body's functions. Depending on the dose, their effects can range from calming down a very nervous person to making a user fall asleep. Depressants are commonly prescribed as legal treatments for people suffering from anxiety (excessive nervousness or worry), high levels of stress, or insomnia.

Some people abuse depressants, however. Common street names for them include barbs, blue devils, downers, jellies, and tranx. All depressants can be dangerous when not taken according to a doctor's instructions. At low doses, depressants produce effects

similar to those of alcohol: mild euphoria, | 25
lightheadedness, and loss of coordination. At
higher doses, depressants can cause problems in thinking, understanding, and
memory; slurred speech; aggressive behavior; and rapid mood changes.

Hallucinogens

Hallucinogens are some of the illegal drugs
most commonly used by teens. This cate-
gory includes LSD (acid), PCP (angel
dust), ecstasy (MDMA), Special K (ketamine hydrochloride), mescaline, and psilocybin, the drug present in shrooms. In
general, hallucinogens strongly affect the
way that users see, hear, feel, touch, and
taste. When high on hallucinogens, users
often lose track of time and place and have
a hard time telling the difference between
the real world and what they are imagining.

Hallucinogens cause insomnia, an
increase in blood pressure and heart rate,
and impairment of muscle coordination
and pain awareness. As a result, users may
put themselves and others in danger by
taking extreme risks or by acting violently
or in unexpected ways. The effects of hallu-
cinogen use are highly unpredictable and
can last for up to twelve hours. In addition,
both LSD and PCP can lead to flashbacks

26 | days, weeks, or even years after drug use.

Special K (ketamine hydrochloride) and ecstasy (MDMA) are two hallucinogens that are becoming increasingly popular among teens. They are often the drugs of choice at raves (all-night underground dance parties) because they keep users feeling happy and energized throughout the night. Special K and ecstasy cause intense hallucinations and distortion of the senses.

Heroin

Heroin, along with opium, morphine, and codeine, is an opiate. The main characteristic of opiates is that they are painkillers. Heroin, the most addictive of the opiates, is usually injected with a needle into the veins (called mainlining), although some people inject it underneath the skin (known as skin-popping). Some common street names for heroin are smack, junk, dope, and brown sugar.

When injected intravenously (into the veins), heroin is absorbed very quickly and causes an immediate rush, an extremely pleasurable feeling that lasts for less than a minute. Users then experience feelings of calmness and well-being, become less nervous and aggressive, and are numb to emotional pain.

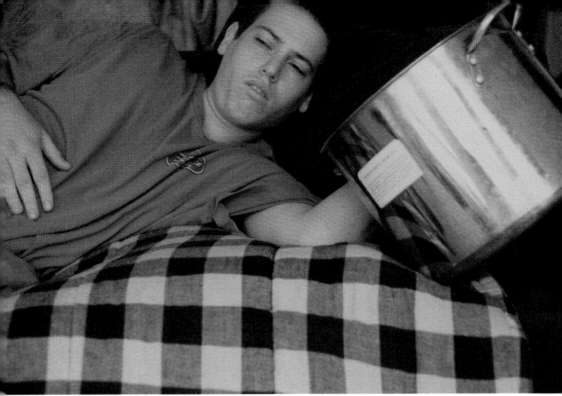

Nausea is one of the many unpleasant effects of heroin use.

Unpleasant effects of heroin use include nausea, restlessness, vomiting, constipation, low blood pressure, and sweating. The most dangerous direct effect of heroin is respiratory depression, in which the user's breathing slows down dramatically, sometimes to the point of death. Long-term use of heroin can lead to irregular menstrual periods, cramping, severe shaking, and unconsciousness.

Heroin use is currently on the rise among young Americans. Nearly 90 percent of heroin users today are under twenty-six, and over 2 percent of high-school seniors in 1998 admitted to using it.

28 | ## *Inhalants*

Inhalants are substances that are sniffed, or inhaled through the nose. Most of the inhalants taken today were never meant to be used as mind-altering drugs. Among the most popular products are gasoline, model airplane glue, nail polish remover, and lighter fluid, as well as many cleaning products.

Short-term effects of inhalants include euphoria, lightheadedness, and intense fantasies, as well as nausea, drooling, sneezing and coughing, slowed reflexes, and impaired muscular coordination. Some users who feel very powerful when high on inhalants may take extreme risks that they would never attempt when sober.

Over time, inhalant use is extremely harmful to the body and brain. It can cause liver and kidney damage, problems with bone formation, and severe mental impairment.

Marijuana

In 1997, nearly one in ten people between the ages of twelve and seventeen used marijuana. Almost half of the twelfth-graders interviewed for a 1998 study reported having tried it. That makes marijuana the most popular drug among teens. Commonly known as pot, grass, and weed,

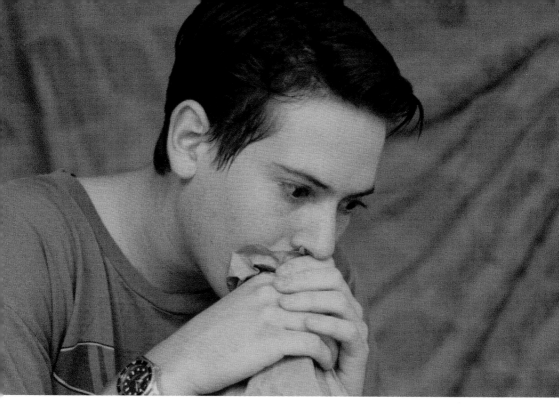

Over time, inhalant use is extremely harmful to the body and brain.

marijuana is usually smoked, though people sometimes swallow it in the form of specially-prepared cookies or brownies.

A typical marijuana high involves mild euphoria, feelings of relaxation and dreaminess, distortion of time and place, and rapid mood changes. Marijuana also increases the heart rate and often causes paranoia and short-term memory loss.

Long-term use of marijuana can badly damage the respiratory system, leading to breathing problems and lung or mouth cancer. It can also harm the immune system, which protects the body from illness and disease.

CHAPTER 3

Drug-Induced Mental Illness

The previous chapters introduced you to some of the most commonly used drugs and how they affect the body and brain. Now we can begin to examine in more detail the complicated relationship between drugs and mental illness.

According to a recent study conducted by the Alcohol, Drug and Mental Health Administration, 15 percent of Americans abuse drugs. But the figure jumps to 50 percent for the number of Americans with a serious mental illness who abuse drugs. These numbers make it clear that there is a strong connection between drug abuse and mental problems.

Drug-Related Mental Illness
The *DSM-IV* breaks down drug-related

mental disorders into two categories:

substance use disorders and substance-induced disorders. (Since the *DSM-IV* uses the term "substance" instead of "drug," the rest of this chapter will follow *DSM-IV* usage to avoid confusion.) The two substance use disorders are substance addiction and substance abuse, both of which are described in the first chapter of this book. Substance-induced disorders—disorders that are directly caused by the use of drugs—include substance intoxication and substance withdrawal, as well as substance-induced mood, anxiety, and psychotic disorders.

Substance-Induced Disorders

We have already looked at one of the substance-induced disorders, withdrawal (see chapter 1). In general, withdrawal is a change in both behavior and physical health due to the sudden absence of a substance in the body of someone who has been using that substance heavily and over a long period of time.

Intoxication

Intoxication refers to a sudden, serious, harmful psychological change that shows up soon after drug use and goes away over time. Basically, it refers to the state of being high. For instance, if someone takes ecstasy and

32 as a result feels dizzy, nauseous, and panicked. According to the *DSM-IV*, even though this person may be a regular user and her reaction is temporary, her state of intoxication is still considered a mental disorder.

Substance-Induced Mood Disorder

Mood disorders are mental disorders that have a disturbance or change of mood as their major symptom. The two major mood disorders are depression and bipolar disorder, also known as manic depression. We can all be moody at times, switching from happy to angry to sad to disappointed over the course of a few hours. Teens in particular often experience frequent mood swings as a result of the many hormonal changes going on in their bodies.

But mood disorders are much more serious than having an occasional moody day. People who suffer from a mood disorder experience significant distress or impairment for at least two weeks in their functioning at home, work, or school, as well as in social situations with friends or family.

Like general mood disorders, substance-induced mood disorder is defined as a mental
32 state in which a strong and ongoing mood

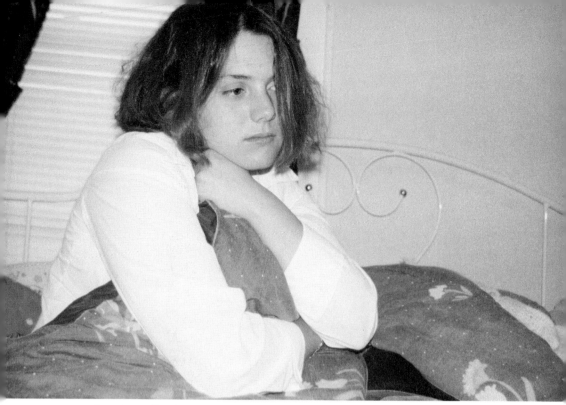

People who suffer from a mood disorder experience significant distress or impairment for at least two weeks.

disturbance causes significant distress and impairment at home, work, or school. The difference is that in substance-induced mood disorder, the mood disturbance is directly due to the physical effects of a drug. There are three subtypes of substance-induced mood disorder. The subtype a person is diagnosed with depends on the nature of his or her main mood disturbance, which is characterized either by depression or irritability or by an unusually elevated level of excitement.

- ***Substance-Induced Mood Disorder with Depressive Features***
  This subtype describes people whose primary symptoms are similar to those

34 | of a major depressive episode: feelings of worthlessness, hopelessness, extreme sadness, excessive guilt, or irritability; lack of interest or pleasure in most activities; significant weight loss or gain; sleeping problems; lack of energy or interest in sex; trouble concentrating or thinking; and frequent thoughts about death or suicide.

- ***Substance-Induced Mood Disorder with Manic Features*** People with this diagnosis show symptoms that strongly resemble a manic episode: excessive self-esteem or grandiosity (a false feeling of being very important and powerful), increased energy, decreased need for sleep, talkativeness, racing thoughts (ideas that fly by too fast for others to follow), distractibility, poor judgment, and denial that anything is wrong.

- ***Substance-Induced Mood Disorder with Mixed Features*** This subtype is used if the symptoms of both mania and depression are present, but neither predominates.

Substance-Induced Anxiety Disorder

Like mood disorders, anxiety disorders involve feelings that we all have, but to an

extreme degree. All of us have felt butter- |
flies in our stomach before a performance, a speech, or even a date. However, people with an anxiety disorder are so nervous and stressed that they cannot deal with the events of daily life.

Four of the major anxiety disorders are generalized anxiety, panic, phobias, and obsessive-compulsive disorder. Subtypes of substance-induced anxiety disorder can produce symptoms similar to the symptoms of all four of these disorders.

- ***Substance-Induced Anxiety Disorder with General Anxiety*** The major characteristic of this subtype resembles the main symptom of general anxiety disorder (GAD): excessive worry and anxiety that is difficult or impossible to control. Other common symptoms of GAD that may be present in the substance-induced form are restlessness, being tired, difficulty concentrating, irritability, muscle tension, and sleep problems.

- ***Substance-Induced Anxiety Disorder with Panic Attacks*** Panic attacks can occur as part of several different anxiety disorders. A panic attack is a specific period of time during which the person feels intense

36

fear or discomfort. The attack usually begins very suddenly and reaches its peak very quickly (usually in ten minutes or less) and is often accompanied by a feeling of future danger and an urge to escape. In addition, at least four out of the following thirteen symptoms must occur for someone to be diagnosed with a panic attack: pounding heart or rapid heartbeat, sweating, shaking, shortness of breath, the feeling of choking, chest pain, nausea or stomach pains, feeling dizzy or lightheaded, feelings of being unreal or being detached from oneself, fear of going crazy, fear of dying, numbness or tingling, and chills or hot flashes.

• ***Substance-Induced Anxiety Disorder with Phobic Symptoms*** A phobia is defined in the *DSM-IV* as a marked, persistent, and unreasonable fear of clearly identifiable objects or situations, such as snakes or spiders, large dogs, needles, being high up, or being in tunnels or on bridges. People with phobias get frightened to a degree that is very much out of proportion to the supposed threat. They realize and admit that their fear is unreasonable and excessive, but they cannot control their reactions to the event or object that causes their fear.

• *Substance-Induced Anxiety Disorder with Obsessive-Compulsive Symptoms* The main features of obsessive-compulsive disorder are repetitive obsessions or compulsions that take up large amounts of time (more than one hour a day) or cause significant distress or impairment in day-to-day life. Obsessions are thoughts, images, or ideas that the person cannot control and cannot get out of his or her head. The person feels very anxious and upset about having these thoughts, which most commonly involve a fear of contamination (getting dirty or infected), a need to keep things in a very specific order (such as keeping objects on a shelf exactly in the same position), aggressive or horrifying impulses (such as a sudden urge to attack a young child), and sex-related images. People who suffer from obsessions develop compulsions— repetitive behaviors or mental acts— as an attempt to get rid of the stress caused by their obsessions. Typical

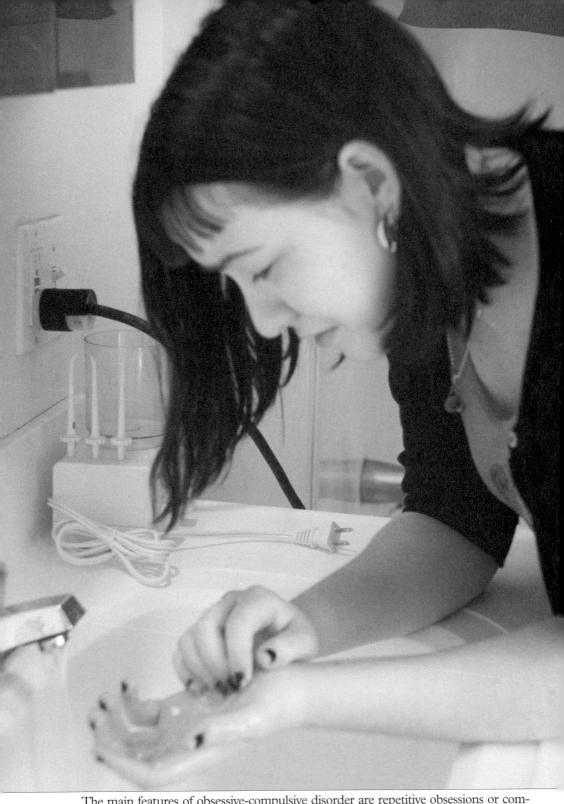

The main features of obsessive-compulsive disorder are repetitive obsessions or compulsions (such as hand washing) that cause significant distress or impairment.

compulsions include praying, count-
ing, repeating words again and again
silently, washing the hands over and
over, arranging objects in order, or
checking many times to make sure
that the stove is turned off or that
the door is locked.

Substance-Induced Psychotic Disorder

The main features of substance-induced
psychotic disorder are strong hallucinations
or delusions, or both, that are due to the
direct effects of a drug. Hallucinations are
imagined sights, sounds, tastes, or smells
that the person believes are real. An
example would be hearing voices that seem
to be near you, but that no one else around
you can hear. Delusions are extremely
strong false beliefs that a person holds on
to even when there is a lot of evidence that
the belief is false. A common delusion is
thinking that you are a famous person, like
the president of the United States or the
rock star Marilyn Manson.

Hallucinations can occur as an effect of
many kinds of drugs, such as alcohol,
amphetamines, inhalants, heroin, and
hallucinogens. But a person is diagnosed
with substance-induced psychotic disorder,
instead of just intoxication, only if he or she

40 does not realize that the hallucinations are connected with drug use. For example, let's say that someone is high on LSD and starts to imagine thousands of ants crawling up his or her legs. If the person knows that the ants are not real and that the vision is a result of using LSD, his or her condition would not be considered substance-induced psychotic disorder. To be diagnosed as psychotic, someone has to be out of touch with reality, unable to tell what is real and what is a creation of his or her imagination. To a psychotic person, the ants are real and have nothing to do with using drugs.

CHAPTER 4

Teens, Drugs, and the Mind

Which Comes First?

So far we have looked at a variety of mental illnesses listed in the *DSM-IV* that are caused by drug use. But in reality, it can be very difficult for parents, friends, and doctors to determine whether a person actually became mentally ill as a result of drug use, or whether the mental illness came first and led the person to begin taking drugs. Accurate diagnosis is especially difficult—and especially important— for teenage patients, since both mental disorders and substance use frequently have their onset (beginning) during the teen years. The earlier a problem is identified correctly and treated, the better the chance of recovery.

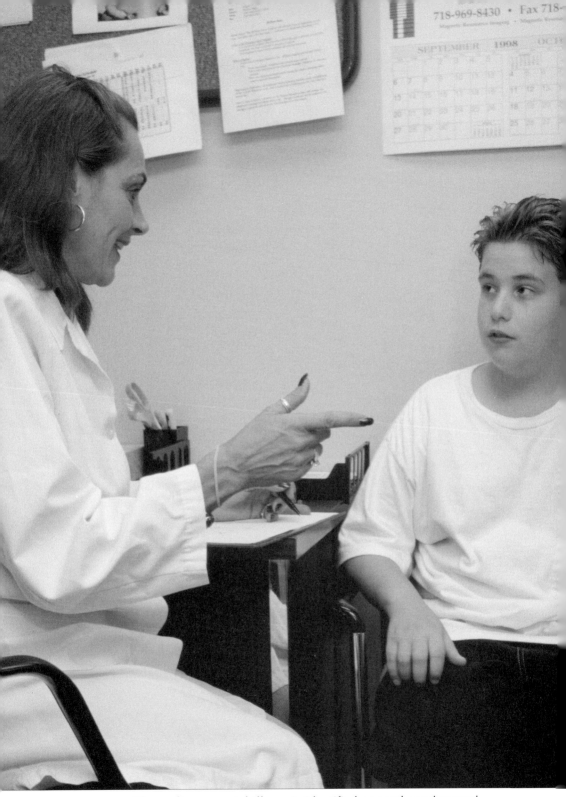

The earlier a mental illness is identified correctly and treated,
the better the chance of recovery.

Symptoms of drug use can often mask an underlying mental problem, leading doctors to treat mentally ill patients for their drug abuse problems but not for their more serious mental illness. A related problem is that the effects of many drugs mimic (closely resemble) the symptoms of common mental illnesses; for example, large doses of sedative-hypnotics can make people seem temporarily depressed, and amphetamines can lead to a manialike state.

Why Do Teens Use Drugs?

The teen years can be pretty rough. You may feel as if your parents do not understand you and that you do not fit in with your friends. Maybe school seems like a drag and you are looking for some excitement. You probably also feel insecure about yourself sometimes, especially with all the physical and mental changes that you are going through. All of these feelings make it easy to let peer pressure, the desire to rebel against authority, or even just a wish for adventure, take control even when you know that you should stay away from drugs. Experts have several theories about which factors lead teens to try drugs and why.

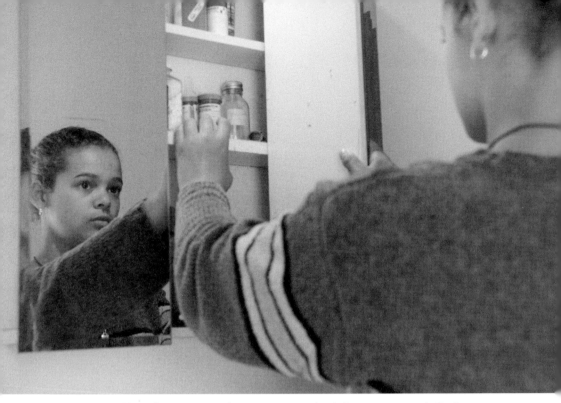

Self-medicating, or taking nonprescribed drugs, is a quick fix for emotional problems that can actually lead to more serious mental illness.

Self-Medication

People in our society often look for quick fixes for their problems. Drugs can seem like an easy way for teens to get rid of bad feelings or to fulfill an emotional need. Taking nonprescribed drugs as an attempt to escape from problems is called self-medication.

A related explanation for the link between mental illness and street drug use in teens is that people who are in the process of developing a mental illness such as depression, schizophrenia, or panic disorder sometimes turn to mind-altering drugs to explain the experiences that they

are having. Taking a mind-altering drug like | **45**
marijuana or LSD can give the person a
possible explanation for his or her hallucinations—it's the drugs, not me.

Disinhibition

As a teen, you are trying to figure out who
you are and where you fit in. Sometimes the
struggle to become your own person, sepa-
rate from your parents, makes you want to
go out and try some wild things that your
parents disapprove of. Disinhibition refers to
the feeling that many teens have that even
though they know something is dangerous or
wrong, they can, and will, do it anyway—no
matter what the consequences are.

Of course, it is not just teens who engage
in risky behaviors just for "fun." There are
plenty of adults who act irrationally or dan-
gerously in search of excitement. But
young people tend to feel that they are
untouchable by death or danger. This fear-
lessness, combined with the wish to rebel
against parents, teachers, and other author-
ities, leads many teens to engage in impul-
sive behaviors, such as trying drugs.

Parental Influence

Studies show that parental influence is a key
factor in determining whether teens end up
using drugs. Teens who are well-supervised by

46 | their parents and who feel that their parents care about them are less likely to use drugs than teens whose parents pay less attention to them. If a teen does not find support and love at home, he or she will seek it from friends. This will make the teen more likely to go along with the crowd to keep friendships strong. As a general rule, the group of teens most likely to use drugs are those who have troubled family relationships or whose parents are drug users.

What Goes Up Must Come Down

According to a 1999 study, adolescents with emotional problems were nearly four times more likely to be addicted to drugs or alcohol than other adolescents, and nearly seven times more likely to have used illegal drugs in the past month.

If you or someone you know is considering using drugs to get rid of feelings like anger, sadness, or even just boredom, remember: Drugs only make things worse. You may feel relaxed and far away during your high, but you always come back down—and when you do, the problems are still there.

Find other ways to express your feelings and to have fun. Try out many different activities until you find one that you like, and stick with it. Painting, dancing, debating, cooking,

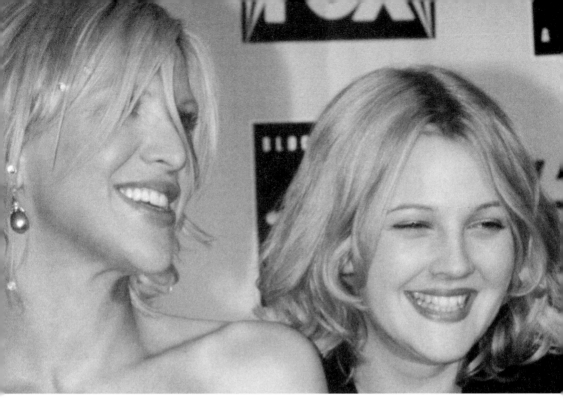

Both Courtney Love and Drew Barrymore have chosen to lead drug-free lives.

hiking, writing, and acting are just a few of the many possibilities. Exercise works for many people. It is cheap, easy, and a very effective way to achieve a natural high.

If you are not into team sports or dislike intense activity, try yoga or martial arts. Courtney Love, lead singer of the rock band Hole, was once famous for using a lot of drugs with her husband, Kurt Cobain, who led the band Nirvana before his death in 1994. Now Love is clean and relies on meditation, exercise, and playing music to work out her problems. Drew Barrymore, another former drug addict, practices yoga to keep healthy and relaxed.

If they can do it, so can you.

CHAPTER 5

Drugs That Help

Medications are one of the most common, and most effective, ways to treat mental conditions today. The first such medication, chlorpromazine, was introduced only forty-one years ago, but since that time vast strides have been made in the field of psychotherapeutics (the use of medicines to treat mental problems). Thousands of people who in the first half of this century might have spent many years in mental hospitals are now able to live and work in their communities with the help of medication.

Cures Versus Treatments

The treatment of a mental illness with drugs can be compared to the treatment of diabetes with insulin. Insulin allows people with diabetes to control their symptoms, but it does not cure diabetes—that is, it does not get rid of the causes of the illness. People with diabetes must continue to take insulin regularly in order to stay healthy.

Similarly, medication allows a person with a mental disorder to control his or her symptoms, but it does not cure the underlying mental condition. If a diabetic stops taking insulin, he or she will get very sick. In the same way, the symptoms of a mental disorder will become much worse if the person stops taking his or her psychotherapeutic drug.

For How Long Are These Drugs Taken?

The length of time that someone must take psychotherapeutic drugs depends on the kind of mental disorder. Someone with depression or anxiety can often take medication for a single period of several weeks or months and then never need the drug again. More serious conditions, such as manic depression and schizophrenia, require regular medication use, usually for many years.

How Much of the Drug Is Needed?

Like all medications, psychotherapeutic drugs have different effects on different

50 | people. Some people need more of a medication to experience its helpful effects, whereas others may be sensitive to extremely small doses of the same drug. Side effects can seriously affect some patients and not affect others at all. Some factors that can influence the effects of a medication include age, gender, body size, physical illnesses, eating habits, and cigarette smoking.

What Kinds of Medications Exist?

The most commonly used psychotherapeutic drugs can be grouped into four main categories: antidepressant, antianxiety, antimanic, and antipsychotic medications. As their names suggest, these medications treat symptoms of depression, anxiety, mania, and psychotic disorders, respectively.

Antidepressant Medications

Antidepressants are used to help control the symptoms of both depression and anxiety disorders. For people with depression, antidepressants reduce or remove feelings of sadness, guilt, and fatigue, and help the person feel more like he or she did before the depression set in. Patients with anxiety use antidepressants to block the symptoms of panic, such as rapid heartbeat, dizziness, nausea, and breathing problems.

There are three major categories of anti-depressants: tricyclic antidepressants, MAOIs (monoamine oxidase inhibitors), and SSRIs (selective serotonin reuptake inhibitors). Both tricyclics and MAOIs have far more dangerous side effects than SSRIs. Tricyclic antidepressants, which are used for very serious cases of depression, can cause blurred vision, weight gain, muscle twitches, and weakness, and can interact with many common drugs, such as birth control pills, aspirin, and tobacco. MAOIs are used to treat cases of depression that involve unusual symptoms like panic attacks and phobias. Possible side effects of MAOIs include dizziness, rapid heartbeat, and very dangerous interactions with certain foods and alcoholic drinks as well as medications. These interactions can cause severe high blood pressure, vomiting, psychosis, seizures, and coma. MAOI users must make sure to get a list from their doctor of foods, drinks, and medicines to avoid.

SSRIs are some of the most popular, well-advertised, and well-tolerated drugs used today. Prozac, Zoloft, Paxil, Effexor, and Luvox are all SSRIs. They work very

52 | differently from MAOIs and tricyclic antidepressants, and in general have far fewer and far less dangerous side effects. The most common complaints of SSRI users are stomach problems and headaches, although some people experience more troubling effects, such as sleeping problems, anxiety, and a loss of sexual interest. SSRIs are usually used to treat less serious cases of depression and can also be used to help patients—like Darnell in this book's introduction—to overcome an eating disorder like anorexia or bulimia.

Antianxiety Medications

Antianxiety medications help to calm and relax anxious patients and to remove anxiety symptoms such as panic, uneasiness, stomachache, breathing problems, and rapid heartbeat. There are several kinds of antianxiety drugs in use today. The preferred type are the benzodiazepines, such as Xanax and Valium. Like barbiturates, benzodiazepines are sedative-hypnotic drugs that slow down the central nervous system. Doctors prefer to prescribe benzodiazepines because they are milder and less addictive than barbiturates.

Benzodiazepines act fast. Most begin to work within a few hours, and some act even

more rapidly. They have few side effects, *53*
but they can lead to drowsiness, loss of coordination, and, occasionally, mental confusion and fatigue. For these reasons, it can be dangerous to drive or operate machinery while using these medications, especially for people who are just beginning treatment. In addition, the interaction between benzodiazepines and alcohol can lead to serious and even fatal consequences, so it is best to avoid drinking alcohol when taking these drugs. Benzodiazepines can also interact with antihistamines (allergy medications), anesthetics (drugs that numb the body), and certain prescription pain medications, so it is especially important to follow the doctor's instructions on what substances to avoid.

Antimanic Medications

Mania can occur as a symptom of a number of mental disorders, but it is most commonly associated with manic depression, also known as bipolar disorder. People with manic depression shift between periods of extremely "low" moods (the depressive states) and extremely "high" moods (the manic periods).

When someone is in a manic high, he or she may be overactive, extremely talkative,

54 excessively energetic, and may tend to jump quickly from one topic to another. Other people often cannot keep up with the person's words, ideas, or actions. People who are manic are frequently irritable, are easily distracted, and have very grand ideas about themselves and what they can achieve. This can lead to huge shopping sprees, out-of-control sex or drug use, or other reckless behaviors that they regret greatly later when their mania disappears.

The most commonly used antimanic drug is lithium, which usually begins to reduce manic symptoms in about five to fourteen days. Since lithium acts to even out both the low and the high mood swings, it is used not just to treat severe manic attacks, but as an ongoing treatment for manic depression. When first using lithium, a patient can experience side effects, including drowsiness, weakness, vomiting, trembling, increased thirst, and weight gain. An additional problem with lithium treatment is that the amount that a person must take to benefit from the drug is very close to the amount that is toxic to humans. For this reason, lithium users need to check the amount of lithium in their blood every few months to make sure that it does not reach a toxic level.

Antipsychotic Medications

Someone who is psychotic is out of touch with the real world. He or she may hallucinate, have delusions, and begin to stop taking care of him- or herself. Often severely psychotic individuals will stop bathing and changing clothes, say things that make no sense, and spend most of their time alone. Psychosis can occur with several mental disorders, including very severe depression and extreme cases of mania, but it is most commonly associated with a mental illness called schizophrenia.

Antipsychotic medications, also known as neuroleptics, take away these symptoms or make them milder. There are several kinds of neuroleptics, including Thorazine and Haldol. Most of the side effects are mild.

Use with Caution!

Like all drugs, psychotherapeutic medications must be taken exactly as the doctor prescribes them. Users should be very careful to avoid all foods, drinks, and other substances that may interact with the drug, and should know the warning signs of dangerous interactions or incorrect dosages. Other things to be aware of include possible side effects, the name

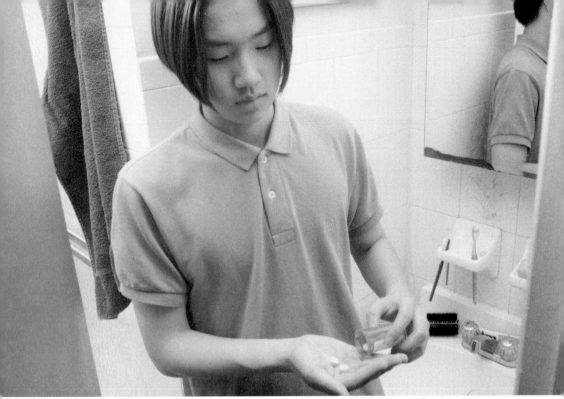

When taking medication you should be aware of the various side effects that the drug may cause.

and purpose of the medication, and the proper way to use it.

Reaching Out

If you think that you or someone you know needs help with drug-related problems or with mental problems—or both—it is vital to get support. Reading books like this one is a good first step in finding out more about drugs and mental illness, but it is up to you to follow through and get help.

Glossary
Explaining New Words

central nervous system The part of the nervous system consisting of the brain and the spinal cord.

coma A state of deep unconsciousness from which a person cannot be roused; caused by disease or injury.

convulsion An uncontrollable and extremely strong contraction of the muscles.

delusion An extremely strong false belief that a person holds on to even when there is a lot of evidence that the belief is false.

flashback An unexpected and usually brief return of the effects of a hallucinogenic drug long after its original use.

58 | **hallucination** Imagined sights, sounds, tastes, or smells that the person believes are real but that have no identifiable stimulus (cause).

impairment Diminishment, as in strength or ability.

joint A slang term for a marijuana cigarette.

mescaline (peyote) A hallucinogenic drug found on the tops of a certain kind of cactus.

neurons Cells in the brain and spinal cord that act as messengers between the body and the brain.

paranoia An unrealistic and extreme suspicion or distrust of others.

schizophrenia A serious illness that affects the brain and causes major problems with thinking, emotions, and behavior.

seizure A sudden attack or convulsion, usually due to a physical disorder or to drug use.

upper A slang term for stimulants, especially amphetamines.

Where to Go for Help

If you need immediate help, call these confidential twenty-four hour hotlines:

Boys Town National Hotline
(800) 448-3000

National Substance Abuse Hotline
(800) DRUG HELP (378-4437)
(800) HELP 111 (435-7111)

Youth Crisis Hotline
(800) HIT HOME (448-4663)

In the United States
Dual Disorders Anonymous
P.O. Box 681264
Schaumberg, IL 60168-1660
(847) 956-1660
National Alliance for the Mentally Ill
200 North Glebe Road, Suite 1015

60 | Arlington, VA 22203-3754
(800) 950-NAMI

In Canada
Canadian Mental Health Association
2610 Yonge Street
Toronto, ON M4S 2Z3
(416) 484-7750

Web Sites
Mental Health InfoSource
http://www.mhsource.com

Mental Health Net
http://mentalhealth.net/guide/substance.ht
m

Mental Wellness.com
http://www.mentalwellness.com

NAMI/NYC
http://www.nami-nyc-metro.org

National Institute of Mental Health
http://www.nimh.nih.gov

Web of Addictions
http://www.well.com/user/woa

For Further Reading

Colvin, Rod. *Prescription Drug Abuse: The Hidden Epidemic*. Omaha, NE: Addicus Books, 1995.

Gorman, Jack M., M.D. *The Essential Guide to Psychiatric Drugs*. New York: St. Martin's Press, 1990.

Graedon, Joe, and Teresa Graedon. *The People's Guide to Deadly Drug Interactions*. New York: St Martin's Press, 1990.

Phillips, Lynn. *Life Issues: Drug Abuse*. New York: Marshall Cavendish, 1994.

Ryan, Elizabeth A. *Straight Talk About Drugs and Alcohol*. New York: Facts on File, 1995.

Ryglewicz, Hilary, A.C.S.W., and Bert Pepper, M.D. *Lives at Risk: Understanding and Treating Young People with Dual Disorders*. New York: The Free Press, 1996.

Index

A

abuse, 8, 10, 19
alcohol, 13, 17–18, 46, 51, 53
physical effects of, 21–22,
    25, 39
Alcohol, Drug and Mental
    Health Administration,
    study by, 30
amphetamines, 18, 22–24,
    39, 43
antianxiety medications, 50,
    52–53
antidepressants, 8, 9, 13,
    50–52
antimanic medications, 50,
    53–54
antipsychotic medications,
    50, 54–55
anxiety, 20, 24, 35, 37, 49,
    50, 52

B

barbiturates, 24, 52
Barrymore, Drew, 47
Benzedrine, 22

benzodiazepines, 24, 52–53
binge drinking, 21

C

caffeine, 14
cellular tolerance, 17–18
chlorpromazine, 48
cocaine, 15, 22–24
compulsions, 16, 37–39
compulsive use, 15, 16
crack, 22
craving, 15, 17, 18

D

delusions, 23, 39, 55
depressants/sedative-hypnotics,
    21, 24–25, 43, 52
depression, 16, 32, 33–34,
    43, 44, 49, 50–52, 55
Dexedrine, 22
*Diagnostic and Statistical
    Manual of Mental Dis-
    orders (DSM-IV)*,
    14–15, 30–31, 32, 36, 41
disinhibition, 45

drug/substance abuse, 10,
    14–15, 19, 30, 31, 43
drug/substance addiction, 10,
    14, 15–16, 19, 31, 46
    physical, 16–18
    psychological, 18

E

ecstasy (MDMA), 25–26, 31

G

general anxiety disorder
    (GAD), 35

H

Haldol, 55
hallucinations, 23, 24, 26,
    39–40, 45, 55
hallucinogens, 25–26, 39
heroin, 8–9, 26–27, 39

I

inhalants, 28, 39
insomnia, 16, 23, 24, 25
intoxication, 31–32, 39

L

lithium, 54
Love, Courtney, 47
LSD (acid), 25–26, 40, 45

M

mania, 34, 43, 50, 53–54, 55
manic depression/bipolar
    disorder, 32, 49, 53
marijuana, 7, 28–29, 45
medication, over-the-counter,
    9, 13–14, 20
medication, prescription, 9,
    13, 20, 22, 24, 53
mescaline, 25
monoamine oxidase inhibitors

(MAOIs), 51–52

N

neuroleptics, 55

O

obsessions, 37
obsessive-compulsive
    disorder, 37
opiates, 26

P

panic attacks, 35–36, 51
parental influence, 45–46
PCP (angel dust), 25–26
phobias, 36–37, 51
Prozac, 8, 51
psilocybin, 25
psychosis, 24, 51, 55
psychotherapeutic drugs,
    48–50
    categories of, 50–55

R

recovery, 19, 41

S

schizophrenia, 44, 49, 55
selective serotonin reuptake
    inhibitors (SSRIs),
    51–52
self-medication, 44–45
smoking/nicotine, 13, 21, 50
Special K (ketamine
    hydrochloride), 25–26
stimulants, 21, 22–24
street drugs, 9, 21, 22, 44
stress, 18, 24, 35
substance-induced anxiety
    disorder, 31, 34–39
substance-induced disorders,
    31–40

64

substance-induced mood
    disorder, 31, 32–34
substance-induced psychotic
    disorder, 31, 39–40
substance use disorders, 31

T
Thorazine, 55
tolerance, 15–16
tricyclic antidepressants,
    51–52

V
Valium, 20, 52

W
withdrawal, 15, 16, 31

X
Xanax, 20, 52

About the Author

Maia Miller was born and raised in New York City, where she currently works as a freelance writer and an editor of books for young adults.

Photo Credits

Cover photo and pp. 15, 22, 27, 29, 38, 44 by Christine Walker; p. 2 by Sarah Friedman; pp. 6, 17, 42 by Brian Silak; p. 33 by Les Mills; p. 56 by Bob Van Lindt; p. 47 © The Everett Collection.

Design Layout

Rebecca Stern
Michael Caroleo